ESSENTIAL OILS FOR BEGINNERS

QUICK AND EASY TO UNDERSTAND
ESSENTIAL OIL RECIPES INCLUDED

ETHAN OXFORD

CONTENTS

ESSENTIAL OILS

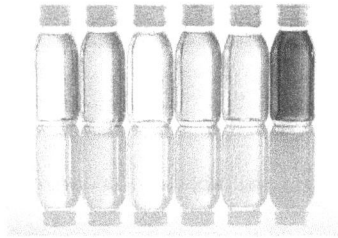

I mportant skin oils are utilized carefully inside aromatherapy and a variety of traditional therapeutic devices. Due to a lot of health benefits involving essential skin oils, they are becoming more and more staying discovered with the scientific neighborhood with regard to the management of various disease which include cancer, HIV, asthma, bronchitis, cardiovascular system cerebral-vascular events, and much more. You can find more than ninety essential skin oils, and just about every provides its very own health benefits. The majority of fat mixture properly with different essential skin oils when it comes to operate and odor, allowing you herbalists to get ready a huge repertoire involving perfumed fat combining.

Underneath will be a summary of essential skin oils that are currently being widespread or reviewed. This skin oil is quite solid inside dynamics which enable it to bring about negative effects which are not taken in a suitable fashion and measure. On top of that, the particular person advantages are generally varied, so that you should check with a new medical doctor ahead of using these types of skin oils, probably contained by or topically. In several personal belongings, the main advantages of your botanical herb will also be furnished inside better depth over an individual web page, therefore think liberal to click on some of people essential skin oils to know the full level involving its health benefits. Here are some of essential oils, involving its health benefits.

Allspice oil

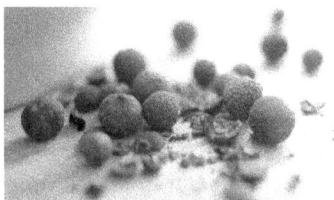

Attributes: It really is considered a great anesthetic, analgesic, antioxidant, antiseptic, carminative, relaxant, stimulant and tonic.

Many benefits: It has been believed for you to cause numbness, reduce pain, relaxes your mind and body, create shade on the pores and skin, and induce many other function.

ANGELICA OIL

A ngelica oil

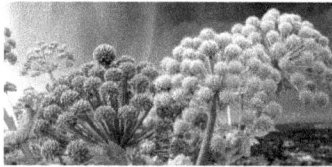

Properties: Angelica oil is typically referred to as a beneficial anti-spasmodic, carminative, depurative, diaphoretic, the digestive system, diuretic, hepatic, expectorant, febrifuge, stimulant, stomachic along with tonic.

Health improvements: That relaxes fits, lower unwanted gas, purifies the bloodstream, advance perspire, help digestion, boost urination, and along with eliminate toxic compound. Angelica oil can also be good for the liver organ, the item relieve obstructed menstruation, expel phlegm & catarrh, lower fever, solution tense ailment, is designed for the belly, also it tone the body.

Anise oil

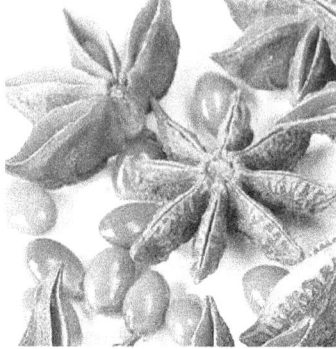

Properties: Usually, it's been utilized as a possible anti-epileptic, anti-hysteric, anti-rheumatic, antiseptic, anti-spasmodic, aperients, carminative, friendly, decongestant, the digestive system, expectorant, insecticide and sedative.

Health improvements: It is frequently currently employed to treat rheumatism & force away septic, rest fits, work as a new purgative, take out unwanted gas, cozy the entire body, clear congestion, along with simplicity inhaling and exhaling. Furthermore, a number of users use anise gas to facilitate digestion, discharge phlegm & catarrh, eliminate & repel insects, red worms along with lice, along with to cure tense conditions.

Basil oil

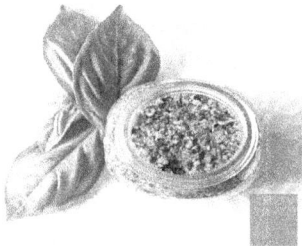

Properties: Basil gas is carminative, anti-spasmodic, analgesic, and antibacterial, along with ophthalmic.

Health improvements: That is definitely used for skin care, respiratory system problem, attack, tension ailment, the circulation of blood problem, discomfort, along with sickness.

BAY OIL

Properties: It's utilized while antiseptic, antibiotic, anti-neuralgic, anti-spasmodic, analgesic, astringent, febrifuge, insecticide, sedative and stomachic.

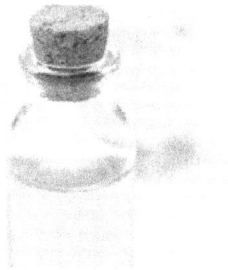

Health improvements: bay oil protect versus septic, prevent microbial development, allow relief from neuralgia discomfort, relaxes fits, provide pain relief, boost urge for food, tighten gums & muscle tissue along with allow quit hair thinning. Different purpose have been pertaining to the treating hemorrhage, marketing regarding bile release, pain relief regarding obstructed menstruation, along with decline regarding fever. The main essential oil additionally will kill & repel insect, sedate inflammation & tense condition, along with is designed for the belly, even though escalating perspire & the elimination regarding unwanted toxic compound in the body.

BENZOIC ESSENTIAL OIL

B enzoic essential oil

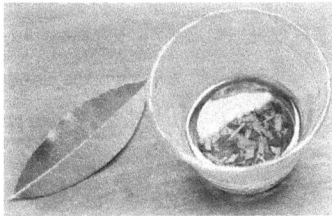

Qualities: It truly is regarded an antidepressant, carminative, good, deodorant, disinfectant, relaxant, diuretic, expectorant, antiseptic, vulnerary, astringent, anti inflammatory, anti-rheumatic along with sedative.

Benefits: That is great for beneficial mood along with fighting major depression, and possesses also been popularized regarding eradicating gasoline build-up, increased temperature your breathing, decreasing human body odor, treating attack, relaxation, advertising urination as well as the succeeding elimination connected with human body harmful toxin. This valuable essential oil likewise strengthens gum along with stop continuous loss of, solution redness, enhances movement and may help cure joint disease, even though comforting nervousness along with reduces stress.

BERGAMOT ESSENTIAL OIL

B ergamot essential oil

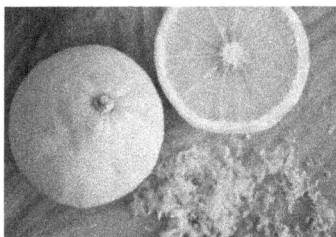

Qualities: It truly is regarded deodorant, vulnerary, antibiotic, antiseptic, anti-spasmodic, sedative, analgesic, antidepressant, disinfectant, febrifuge, along with digestive throughout dynamics.

Benefits: Bergamot essential oil remove human body odor, reduce spasm, depresses pain, enhance disposition along with spat major depression, mend reduce along with scar, along with stimulate useful digestion of food.

Birch essential oil

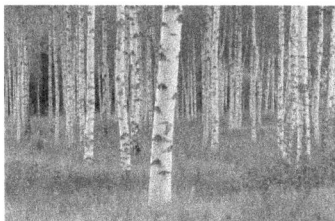

Qualities: It's a tonic, disinfectant, stimulant & antidepressant, analgesic and detoxifier. Moreover, it is a diuretic, germicide and a depurative

Benefits: Birch essential oil spat major depression, lower pain, stimulate urination, protect pain by becoming septic, lower a fever, eliminate germ, along with purifies your our blood.

Bitter almond essential oil

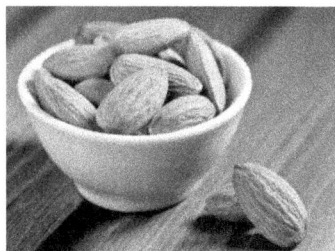

Qualities: It truly is usually applied as being a febrifuge, bactericide, germicide, fungicide, sedative, anesthetic, aperients, diuretic, anti-intoxicant, antispasmodic, so that as a cure for hydrophobia.

Benefits: Your utilize connected with unhealthy almond essential oil are extensively ranged, and will include getting rid of red wiggler, decreasing a fever, getting rid of microorganism, germ along with fungi, sedation along with decreasing redness. Additionally, it may trigger numbness along with become an anesthetic or maybe desensitizing broker. It truly is purgative, increase urination along with assist take away surplus drinking water, sodium, harmful toxin, along with fat in the human body, even though countering the effect connected with intoxicant, treating spasm, along with helping cure hydrophobia, a concern with drinking water, in most case introducing per se throughout somebody who has been infected with rabies.

BLACK PEPPER ESSENTIAL OIL

B lack Pepper essential oil
Qualities: It truly is regarded some sort of digestive, diaphoretic, carminative, antispasmodic, antibacterial, along with an antioxidant.

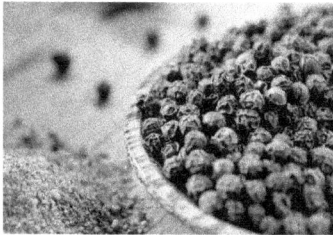

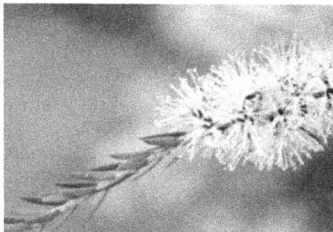

Benefits: This essential oil help with digestion of food,

increase perspiration along with assist take away harmful toxin in the human body. It also aid you to take away un wanted gas in the digestive tract along with won't let these individual increase, even though acting as being a purgative, treating spasm, along with helping treat joint disease along with rheumatism simply by doing away with uric acid and also other harmful toxin in the human body. Dark-colored spice up essential oil inhibit microbial growth; spat early ageing along with neutralize cost-free radical in which deterioration the entire body throughout plenty of mean.

CAJUPUT OIL

C ajuput oil

Qualities: It is common just as one antiseptic, bactericide, expectorant, carminative, and stimulant.

Health advantages: It defend injuries by turning into septic, protect pore and skin, eliminate microbe in addition to pesky insect, solution over-crowding inside the breathing, lower soreness, solution cough, lower nausea, solution spasm, and provide respite from the soreness connected with neuralgia. Cajuput oil additionally take away fume, stimulate secretion in addition to sensation problem replies, tone upward normal technique, boost perspire, offer respite from clogged menses in addition to manage consistent menstruation.

Calamus oil

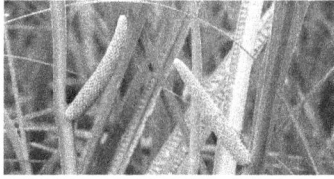

Qualities: It is commonly learn just as one ant rheumatic, antispasmodic, cephalic, circulatory stimulant, memory booster, stimulant in addition to being the tranquilizer.

Health advantages: Calamus oil pleasure rheumatism in addition to osteoarthritis, relaxes spasm, stop microbial expansion, even though being perfect for as their pharmaceutical counterpart in addition to memory. Moreover, the item boost blood vessels & lymph flow, solution tense issues, which enable it to generate sleep.

Chamomile oil

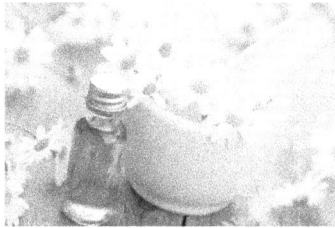

Qualities: Ordinarily, chamomile oil has become used by almost anything you can imagine, which includes their employ just as one antispasmodic, antiseptic, antibiotic, antidepressant, ant neuralgic, carminative, analgesic, febrifuge, hepatic, sedative, digestive system, tonic, bactericidal, stomachic, anti-inflammatory, anti-infectious, in addition to vulnerary.

Health advantages: Chamomile oil may heal fits, guard injuries by turning into septic in addition to corrupted, curb biotic expansion in addition to transmission, struggle depression symptom in addition to uplift disposition, heal neuralgic soreness simply by reducing irritation inside the affected wreck, in addition to soothe redness by nausea. What's more, it reduce fume, encourage release connected with bile, facilitate lessen presence connected with surgical mark, open upward clogged menses in addition to manage all of them, solution soreness, lower nausea, in addition to is useful for the liver organ.

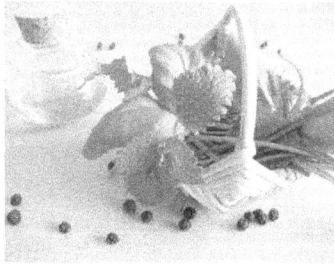

Moreover, chamomile oil sedate redness in addition to hyper-reaction, improve tense system health and fitness, assist digestion of food, lower fits, eliminate microbe, boost perspire, improve digestion of food, in addition to combat transmission. It is just about the most widely used in addition to valuable essential natural oils on the market!

Camphor oil

Qualities: It is a stimulant, antispasmodic, antiseptic, decongestant, anesthetic, sedative, sensation problems pacifier, ant neuralgic, anti-inflammatory, and disinfectant, in addition to a great insecticide.

Health advantages: Camphor oil stimulate solution fits,

defend injuries by transmission, reduce over-crowding, desensitize in addition to function because nearby anes-thetic, calm tense disruption, solution neuralgic soreness, soothes redness, combat transmission, and in addition to eliminate pesky insect.

CARAWAY OIL

C araway oil

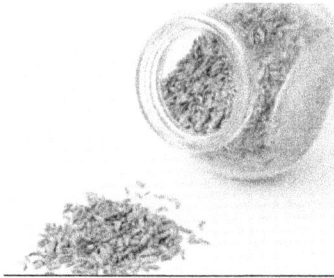

Qualities: It is an antihistaminic, antiseptic, anti spasmodic, carminative, digestive system, stomachic, disinfectant, diuretic, expectorant, aperitif, astringent, insecticide and stimulant.

HEALTH ADVANTAGES: Many experts have seen to raise milk inside the breast, curb histamine to help struggle cough, guard injuries in opposition to turning into septic, and it is good with the coronary heart. Moreover, this particular acrylic solution fits in addition to cramp, take away extra fuel, encourage digestion of food, keep stomach health and fitness, combat transmission, boost urination in addition to facilitate remove poison by system. Ultimately, the item manage menstrual cycle, solution cough, boost urge for food, legal agreement gum in addition to muscle group, eliminate pesky insect, stimulate secretion, and in addition to usually boost overall fitness.

CARDAMOM OIL

C ardamom oil

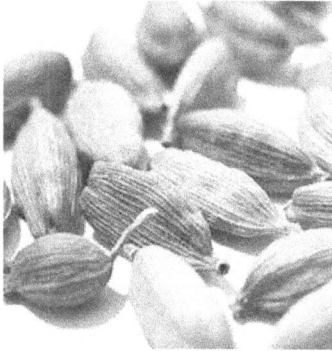

Attributes: It is considered the antispasmodic, and it in addition neutralizes the actual negative effects regarding chemotherapy, lessens nausea. It is utilized being an anti-septic, antimicrobial, stomachic and stimulant, in addition to diuretic agent.

Health advantages: It is often recognized to cure spasm, fight nausea, guard chronic wound in addition to incision, curb microbial expansion, enhance staying power, contract gum, promote digestion, and gaze after abdominal health and fitness. That stimulates secretion along with other capabilities, raises urination in addition to therefore get rid of more salt, bile, h2o, waste in addition to weight on the system.

CARROT SEEDS OIL

C arrot seeds oil

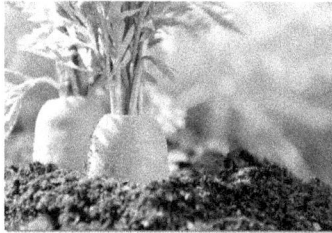

Attributes: It is antiseptic, disinfectant, purifying, anti oxidant, carminative, depurative, diuretic, stimulant, plus a tonic.

Health advantages: Guard chronic wound via growing to be septic, battle transmission, get rid of waste on the system, and neutralize no cost radical in addition to reverse the effect regarding oxidation. Furthermore, the idea get rid of excessive gasoline in addition to doesn't let it develop in the body, while cleaning bloodstream by mean of taking away waste, improving urination, starting in addition to modifiable menses, in adding up to promoting the actual regeneration regarding fresh cellular material.

Cassia oil

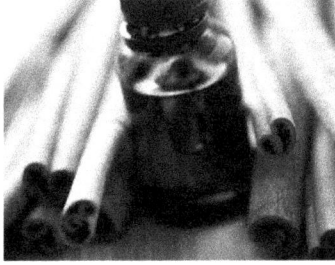

Attributes: It is common being an anti-diarrheal, anti-depressant, antiemetic, antiviral, antimicrobial, and ant rheumatic in addition to the ant arthritic. Other than hundreds of "antis", cassia oil is also the astringent, febrifuge plus a stimulant.

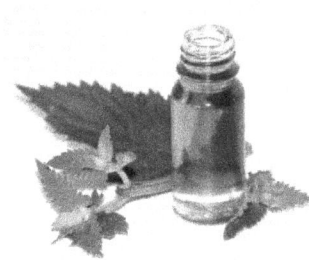

Health advantages: It is often recognizing to remove shed stool in addition to diarrhea, while battling depression symptom in addition to enjoyable spirit. This may also cease nausea, reduce use move, hinder microbial expansion, and take care of rheumatism in addition to joint disease &

muscle group in addition to help stop thinning hair. This specific strong oil is also thought to reduce hemorrhaging, fight virus-like transmission, take away unnecessary gas, advance bloodstream & lymphatic movement, reduce clogged menstruation, in addition to reduce temperature.

CATNIP OIL

C atnip oil
Attributes: This specific less popular acrylic is usually antispasmodic, carminative, diaphoretic, stomachic, stimulant, in addition to astringent.

Health advantages: It is common to fight spasm, take away gases, promote sweating, open up clogged menses in addition to determine the series, strengthen the actual nervous method, preserve abdominal health and fitness, in addition to typically encourage correct method working in the body.

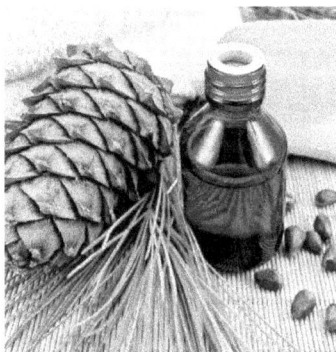

CEDAR WOOD OIL

Cedar wood oil

    Attributes: It is antiseptic, tonic, diuretic, expectorant, sedative, plus a fungicide.

Health advantages: Cedar wood may aid cure chronic wounds, fight spasm, result in contraction inside the gum, muscle group, tissue, skin color in addition to blood vessel, while improving urination and also the succeeding removal regarding waste, h2o, salt in addition to weight on the system. Furthermore, it handle menstrual series, treatment cough in addition to cold, will kill insect pest, and sedate infection in addition to nervous disorder, in addition to stops yeast expansion in addition to transmission.

CINNAMON OIL

C innamon oil

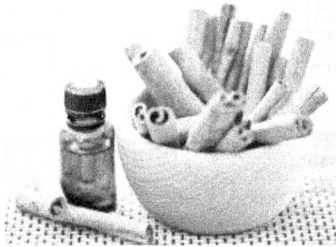

Components: It can be antibacterial, antifungal, antimicrobial, astringent, anti-clotting, revitalizing, a / c, along with carminative within nature.

Health benefits: It can be regularly applied like a mental faculties tonic, and also intended for asthmatic trouble, skin color bacterial infection, blood impurity, the circulation of blood issue, bacterial infection, twisted treatment, alleviation, contraceptive, menstruation trouble, breastfeeding your baby, heart disorder, diabetes, intestinal tract cancer, acid reflux, and as a new pain relief intended for undesirable breath of air!

Citronella oil

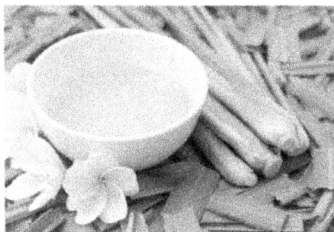

Components: Citronella oil is definitely an antibacterial, anti-inflammatory along with deodorant, just about all rolled straight into just one. It's also diaphoretic, diuretic, fungicidal, stimulant, tonic along with vermifuge. Possibly most well known lately is actually its make use of because a very effective insect pest resistant.

Health benefits: This particular helpful oil prevent microbe, microbial, virus-like & yeast bacterial infection though also killing insect, safeguarding wound coming from getting septic, relaxing inflammation, removing system odor, revitalizing perspiration, improving urination along with the removal of harmful toxin in the system, decreasing nausea, along with repelling insects. Finally, it is good for excellent tummy health and digestive system.

Clary Sage oil

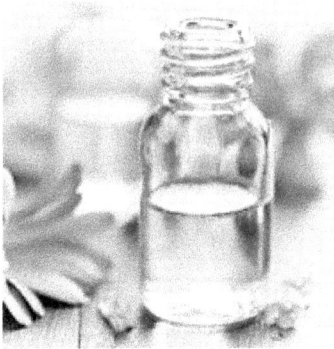

Components: It can be well-known for antidepressant, anticonvulsive, antispasmodic, antiseptic, aphrodisiac, astringent, bactericidal, carminative, deodorant, digestive :, euphoric, hypertensive, sedative, stomachic, along with uterine.

Health benefits: Clary sage oil tiff depression along with uplift mood, stop convulsions by simply sedating stressed disorder, safeguard twisted coming from getting septic, minimize erectile inability along with improve staying power, cause contraction, get rid of bacteria along with curb microbe development. What's more, it removes excess propane, eradicate system odor, help digestive system, lower obstructed menstruation, reduce blood strain, along with create help the health of the stressed technique. Finally, clay sage oil sedate different excessive inner thought along with stress and anxiety, though maintaining excellent tummy health and fixing just about any deterioration sustained with the uterus.

CLOVE OIL

C love oil

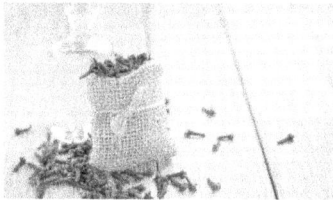

Components: It can be antimicrobial, antifungal, antiseptic, and antiviral, along with revitalizing within nature.

Health benefits: Clove oil is almost certainly found in therapies in connection with dental hygiene, just like toothaches along with cavities, and also intended for bacterial infection, natural skin care, pressure, hassles, asthmatic trouble, earaches, acid reflux, nausea, the circulation of blood issue, blood purification, diabetes, defense mechanism a weakness, premature ejaculation, cholera, along with sties.

Coriander oil

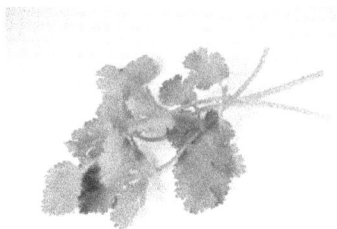

Components: Since then, this specific oil has become used for analgesic, aphrodisiac, antispasmodic, carminative, depurative, deodorant, digestive, fungicide, stimulant, along with stomachic.

Health benefits: It is well-reported to reduce pain, boost staying power, eradicate excess propane, detox the blood, lessen system odor, encourage digestive system, along with hinder yeast development along with infection. Moreover, it minimize extra fat by simply bursting it straight down as a result of hydrolysis, along with maintains a sound body along with strengthen from the tummy.

Cumin oil

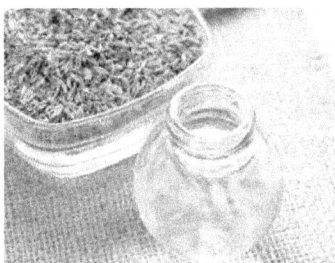

Components: This particular oil is actually bactericidal, carminative, digestive, diuretic, antiseptic, antispasmodic, detoxifying, and stimulant, along with tonic within nature.

Health benefits: It is recognized to get rid of bacteria along with prevent infection, though eliminating excess propane in the bowel, selling digestive system, improving urination, along with safeguarding wound against getting septic. What's more, remove harmful toxin in the blood, oversee the menstrual period, and along with is wonderful for the answer period from the stressed technique.

Cypress oil

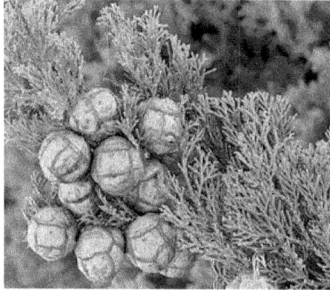

Components: It really is regarded as a astringent, antiseptic, antispasmodic, deodorant, diuretic, hepatic, styptic, vasoconstrictor, asthmatic tonic, plus a sedative.

Benefits: Cypress gas fortifies gum and also legal paper muscle tissue, shield pain in opposition to microbe infection, clear fits, remove entire body scent, will increase urination, advance perspire, fortifies the particular the respiratory system, and also soothes infection.

Coconut Oil

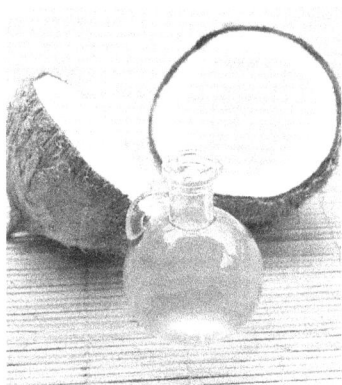

Coconut oil is a palatable oil separated from the portion or meat of developed coconuts gathered from the coconut palm. It has different applications in nourishment, drug, and industry. In light of its high soaked fat substance it is moderate to oxidize and, hence, impervious to acidification, enduring up to two years without ruining.

Benefits of coconut oil

Benefits of coconut oil for hair:

- **Shields Hair Protein**

UNSATURATED FATS TIE to the protein in hair and ensure both the roots and strands of hair from breakage. Lauric corrosive is found in coconut oil and has preferred comes about over other mineral or sunflower oils in the matter of enhancing hair wellbeing.

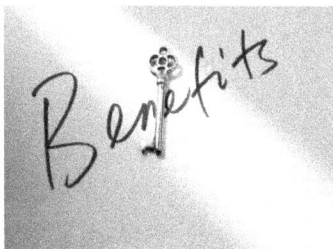

- **Seals in Moisture**

Dampness is vital for sound hair and customary and steady utilization of coconut oil is a valuable method. By entering the hair shaft, coconut oil secures against ecological debasements and abundance heat.

- **Improves Blood Circulation**

A coconut oil scalp back rub will adequately enhance scalp dissemination and support supplement and oxygen conveyance to your hair.

- **Provides Nutrients**

The regular cancer prevention agents and supplements found in coconut oil will convey discriminating assets to enhance your hair's delicateness and gloss. Coconut oil is rich in vitamin E, vitamin K and iron and adequately disposes of dandruff while boosting hair development.

BENEFITS OF COCONUT **oil for skin:**

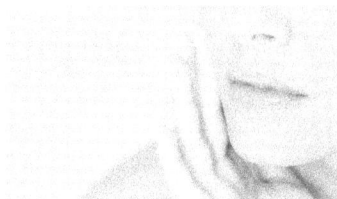

Oil Pulling

In the event that you haven't heard the buzz about oil pulling yet, now is the ideal time to get on the temporary fad. Gargling coconut oil around in your mouth for a day might assist to detoxify your body, whiten teeth, and that's only the tip of the iceberg.

Softening Cuticles

In the event that you wash your hands frequently or your fingernail skin recently require a little T.L.C., apply coconut oil to your fingers twice a day

Soothing Sniffles

Whether you have a runny nose or hypersensitivities, rub a tad of coconut oil inside your nostrils for easing.

Moisturizing Lips

Spread coconut oil over your lips before lights out for hydration that tastes stunning for the duration of the night.

Preventing Wrinkles

Use coconut oil on the range around your eyes to avert wrinkles and under-eye packs.

Treating Acne

Apply coconut oil to imperfections, and abandon it on for around 15 minutes. At that point wash it off with warm water and let your skin air dry (don't have any significant bearing whatever other items). The opposition to bacterial segments in the oil will work to battle skin inflammation.

. . .

OTHER BENEFITS OF COCONUT OIL:

In cooking it work as incredible oil, with a high smoke point. Extraordinary for preparing, mix fries or as a dairy free substitution to spread.

It work as on the skin as an essential cream.

Can help in improving insulin levels

DILL OIL

D ill oil

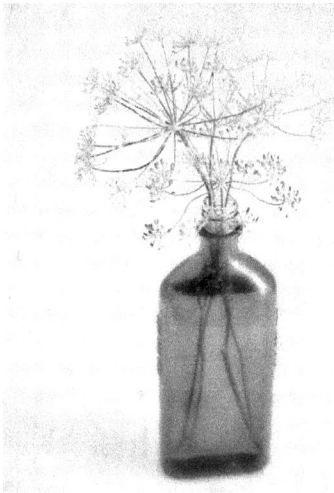

Components: It really is widely used for antispasmodic, carminative, the digestive system, and disinfectant, sedative, stomachic.

Benefits: It really is regularly employed to relieve fits, eliminate extra gas, showcase nutritious food digestion, do not allow microbe infection, improve secretion connected with dairy, calm hypersensitivity and also anxiousness, though currently being good for the particular belly and also growing perspire.

Elemi oil

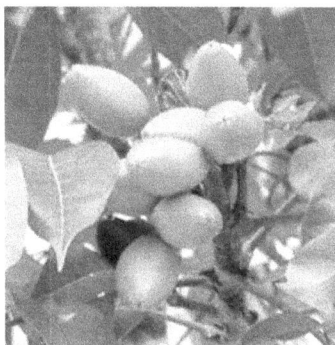

Components: It really is employed for antiseptic, analgesic, expectorant, stimulant and also tonic.

Benefits: It is rather practical with avoiding septic, alleviating agony, expelling phlegm & catarrh, and also usually growing the particular muscles develop and also health on the entire body.

Eucalyptus oil

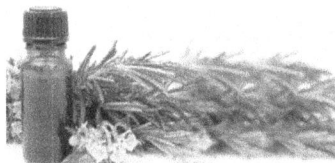

Components: They have numerous essential qualities, which include anti-inflammatory, antispasmodic, decongestant, deodorant, antiseptic, antibacterial, and also stimulating.

Benefits: It is rather practical with treating asthmatic trouble, pain, and muscle agony, thought tiredness, dental care, skincare, diabetes, a fever, and also colon bacteria.

Frankincense oil

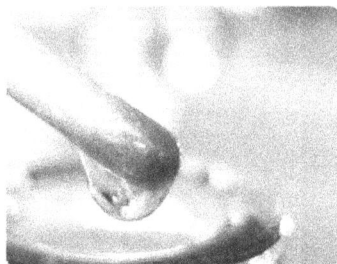

Components: It really is widely used for antiseptic, disinfectant, astringent, and carminative, cicatrizing, the digestive system, and diuretic, expectorant, sedative, tonic, uterine, and also vulnerary.

Benefits: Frankincense oil shield pain coming from getting septic, spat microbe infection, induce contraction with gum, muscle tissue and also leading to tinnitus, and also remove extra gas, cure scarring, maintain cell nutritious and also advance their regeneration.

This advances food digestion, will increase urination, regulates menstrual cycles, programs coughs and also colds, soothes anxiousness and also infection, and also guarantees a sound body on the uterus.

Galbanum oil

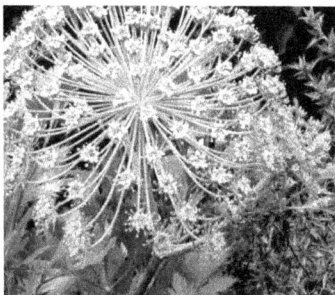

Components: Galbanum oil has turned into engaged for an arthritic, antispasmodic, circulatory stimulant, decongestant, insecticide, ant parasitic plus a vulnerary.

Benefits: Customarily, this goodies rheumatism relaxes spasm, clear scarring and also destinations, will increase our blood and also lymph blood circulation, clear blockage, and also eases breathing. In addition, this removes toxin, help skin tone health, wipe out & repel pesky insect, eliminate parasitic organism, and also quicken the particular curing connected with pains.

GERANIUM OIL

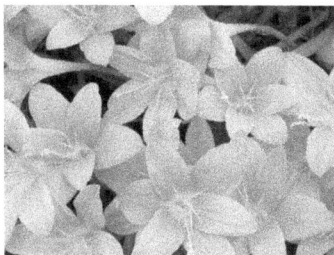

Components: They have a variety of qualities, which include utilize for astringent, haemostatic, cicatrizing, diuretic, deodorant, styptic, tonic, vermifuge, and also vulnerary.

Benefits: It really is currently employed to generate tightening up on the gum, muscle tissue, skin tone and also leading to tinnitus and also with halting hemorrhage, scar tissue curing, campaign connected with cellular increase, and also greater urination. It's also used to quit entire body scent, develop up the entire body, and also kill colon parasitic organisms and also red wigglers.

Ginger oil

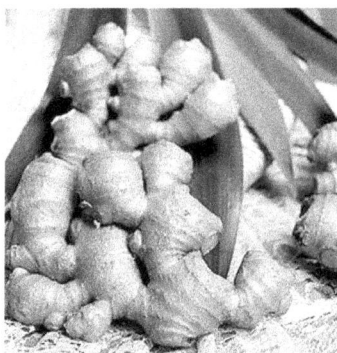

Components: It could be employed for analgesic, antiemetic, antiseptic, antispasmodic, bactericidal, carminative, cephalic, expectorant, febrifuge, laxative, stimulant, stomachic, and also tonic.

Benefits: Ginger oil has become recognized by remedy agony, quit nausea, guard coming from pain getting septic, and also take it easy fits. Some users furthermore use it to prevent microbe increase, eliminate gas, and also enhance brain and also memory space performs, though helping to discharge phlegm & catarrh. Lastly, this is recognized to split fever, crystal clear bowel, deliver coloring to the skin tone, enhance belly health, and also showcase perspiring, which help removes toxin from the entire body.

Grapefruit oil

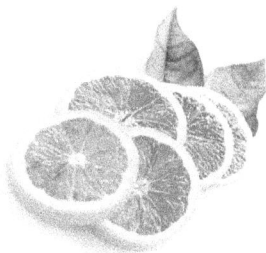

Qualities: This substance is often a diuretic, disinfectant, stimulant, antidepressant, antiseptic, aperitif, lymphatic, and also a tonic.

Many benefits: In a variety of region of the planet, it really is helpful to encourage urination, deal with infection, minimize depression symptom as well as uplift state of mind as well as feeling. Additionally, it shields pain coming from becoming septic even though improving the removal involving toxic compound.

Helicrysum oil

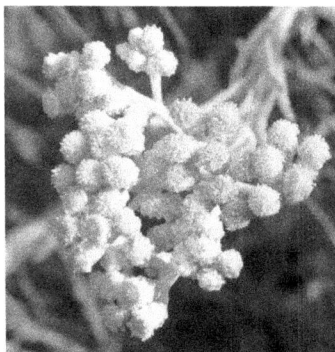

Qualities: This particular oil is antispasmodic, anticoagulant, antiallergenic, antimicrobial, antichloristic, nervine, anti-inflammatory, cicatrizing, expectorant, and febrifuge, anti septic, emollient, fungicidal, hepatic and diuretic.

Many benefits: Individual regularly utilize this fat because doing so lower spasm, keep the fluidity involving blood vessel, combat allergic reaction, check microbial infection, dissolve as well as clear blood vessel clot, lower redness coming from fever, as well as is wonderful for stressed method wellness. Additionally, it lower many other sort of redness, clear phlegm as well as lower cough, mend scar, shield pain coming from becoming septic, influence right bile eliminate into your abdominal, create pore and skin easy as well as youthful, dissolve mucus, as well as eliminate fungus infection. It's also infamously great for the hard working liver as well as spleen, even though stirring urination and also the regeneration involving brand new cellular material.

16

HYSSOP OIL

H yssop oil

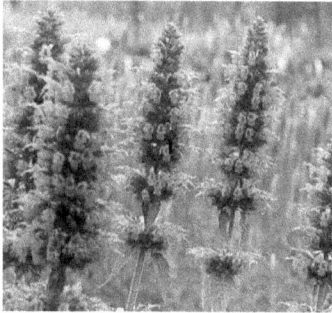

Qualities: Hyssop fat is surely an astringent, stimulant, antispasmodic, ant rheumatic, antiseptic, carminative, cicatrizing, digestive, diuretic, emenagogue, expectorant, hypertensive, nervine, tonic, and febrifuge, vermifuge, vulnerary

Many benefits: The idea induce the tightening up involving gum, muscular tissue, pore and skin as well as arteries and, even though decreasing spasm, removing excess propane, along with advertising speedy healing involving scar as well as after-marks. Additionally, it encourage digestive system, raises urination, handle menstruation, reduce phlegm as well as cough, raise blood vessel force, as well as encourage perspiration. It truly is generally considered to be great for decreasing strain within the stressed method as well as decreasing fever.

17

JASMINE OIL

J asmine oil

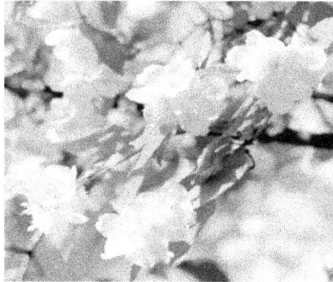

Qualities: It truly is considered an antidepressant, anti-septic, aphrodisiac, antispasmodic, expectorant, emena-gogue, parturient, sedative as well as uterine.

Many benefits: Jasmine oil combat depression symptom as well as uplift feeling, shield pain, solution lovemaking dysfunction, as well as raise sexual desire. Additionally, it lower spasm, mend scar as well as immediately after repre-sent, present rest from phlegm as well as cough, raise bust milk, as well as handle impeded menstrual round. This OIL likewise help reduce the delivery involving infant as well as labor cramping, even though sedating redness as well as stressed disturbance.

Juniper oil

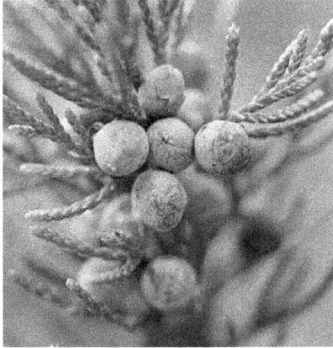

Qualities: Juniper oil is almost certainly referred to as an antiseptic, ant rheumatic, depurative, antispasmodic, stirring, stomachic, astringent, carminative, diuretic and vulnerary as well as tonic.

Many benefits: This particular oil shield pain next to becoming septic, raise perspiration, solution rheumatism as well as joint disease, purifies blood vessel, eliminate spasm, influence characteristics, as well as is wonderful for the abdominal. Juniper fat likewise create gum tougher as well as put a stop to hemorrhaging, lower excess propane, encourage urination, give shade toward the pore and skin, as well as typically encourage speedy healing involving pain.

Lavandin oil

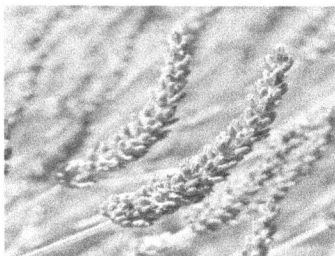

Qualities: It truly is widely used just as one antidepressant, antiseptic, analgesic, expectorant, nervine, as well as vulnerary.

Many benefits: Usually, lavandin fat combat depression symptom, shield pain coming from building infection, lowers ache, mend scar as well as after-mark, clear phlegm as well as solution cough, as well as tone up anxious feeling.

Lavender oil

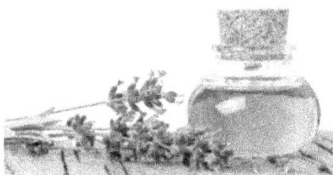

Qualities: Lavender oil might be peaceful, slumber inducting, analgesic, disinfectant, anti-inflammatory, antiseptic, as well as antifungal.

Many benefits: This particular oil is effective for therapy involving problem with the stressed method, sleeping disorder, pain alleviation, urine stream, respiratory issue, healthy skin care, head of hair health care, the circulation of blood, as well as disease fighting capability wellness.

Lemon oil

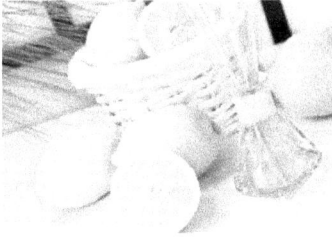

Attributes: lemon oil is usually an antiseptic, and astringent, bactericidal, febrifuge, and restorative, along with a tonic.

Many benefits: This kind of oil protect from acute wound becoming septic, even though inhibiting virus-like and bacterial development, fortifying gum, and halting thinning hair. In addition, it lifting skin, induce tone with muscle group, stop continuous loss of, combat infection, and treatment fever.

Lemongrass oil

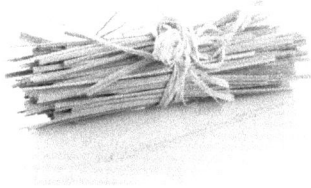

Attributes: It is an analgesic, antidepressant, antipyretic, astringent, bactericidal, carminative, diuretic, insecticidal, and sedative, along with a tonic.

Many benefits: Customarily, lemongrass lessen ache, combat depressive disorder, stops microbial development, lessen substantial vomiting, protect acute wound from getting septic, firm gum and curly hair and lessen continuous loss of. This kind of oil wipe out microorganism, eradicate fuel, lessen system odor, promote urination, lessen vomiting, stop infection, raise dairy, wipe out insect pest, firm anxiety, and soothes irritation and stressed trouble.

Lime oil

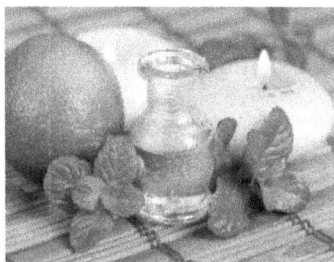

Attributes: Lime scale oil is actually antiseptic, astringent, bactericidal, haemostatic, restorative, and tonic.

Many benefits: This could shield acute wound from becoming septic, control virus-like disease, raise desire for foods, kill microorganism, battle infection, decrease vomiting, quit continuous loss of, and commonly raise wellness.

Mandarin oil

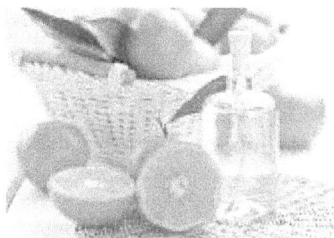

Attributes: It has an antiseptic, antispasmodic, circulatory, depurative, the digestive system, hepatic, stressed relaxant, sedative, stomachic along with a tonic.

Many benefits: This kind of oil protect acute wound toward becoming septic, relaxes spasm, raise body & lymph circulation, promote development & regeneration associated with cellular material, purifies body, encourage digestive function, and is useful for the actual liver. In addition, it soothes irritation and stressed illnesses, even though getting great for the actual tummy and commonly getting fitter one's body.

Manuka oil

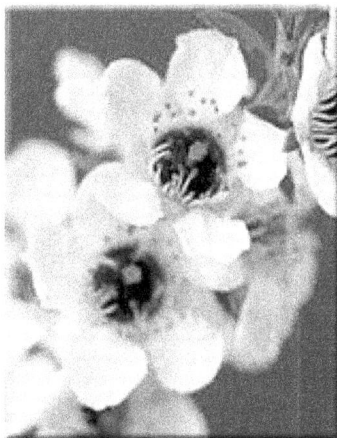

Attributes: Manuka oil is usually antidandruff, an antidote to be able to termite attack and sting, in addition to antibacterial, antifungal, anti-inflammatory, antihistaminic, antiallergenic and deodorant and is a superb stressed relaxant.

Many benefits: It is commonly used to deal with dandruff, table venomous attack, inhibit bacterial and infection, sedate irritation, look at manufacturing associated with histamine and lessen sensitized sign. Lastly, it quickly clear upward mark and area, promote development & regeneration associated with cellular material, and lessen system odor.

Marjoram oil

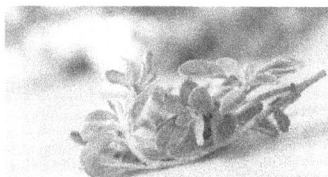

Attributes: Marjoram oil is actually analgesic, antispasmodic, an antiseptic, bactericidal, carminative, cephalic, diaphoretic, the digestive system, expectorant, laxative, stomachic, and vulnerary. Rather the actual active oil!

Many benefits: It is generally given or maybe chosen pertaining to treatment since it lessen ache, eradicate spasm and treatment cramping pain, even though improving the actual sexual desire. Marjoram oil also protect from acute wound becoming septic, stop virus-like and bacterial development, get rid of extra fuel from the intestine, treatment hassles, raise sweat, promote digestive function, raise urination, start up upward blocked menses, treatment cough and cold, and dilute phlegm. Lastly, it could kill fungus, decrease body demand, treat constipation, calm stressed trouble, enlarge and loosen up arteries and, and commonly bettering the healthiness of your tummy.

18

MELISSA OIL

M elissa oil

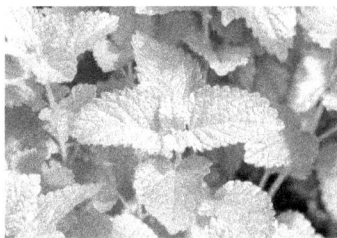

Attributes: It is commonly used as a possible antidepressant, good, nervine, emenagogue, sedative, antispasmodic, stomachic, antibacterial, carminative, diaphoretic, febrifuge, hypertensive, along with a tonic.

Many benefits: Normally, it is utilized as a way to decrease thought associated with depressive disorder, treat stressed disease, wide open clogged menses, sedate irritation, decrease spasm, and is useful for the actual tummy. In addition, it stop microorganism, get rid of fuel, raise sweat & get rid of toxin, even though reducing vomiting, decreasing body demand and increasing the healthiness of your immunity process.

MUGWORT **oil**

Properties: This oil is usually applied as being a friendly, the digestive system, diuretic, emenagogue, nervine, stimulant, uterine, and vermifuge.

Health advantages: Mugwort oil allow for digestion of food, boosts urination and removing regarding toxic compound, pleasure nervous disorder, energize systemic feature, maintain uterine well being, and wipe out abdominal earthworm

19

MULLEIN OIL

M ullein oil

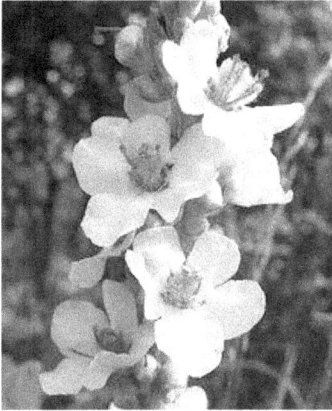

Properties: It really is a good analgesic, anti-inflamma-tory, disinfectant, expectorant, febrifuge, relaxant and tran-quilizing.

Health advantages: It really is regularly employed regarding remedy, and in an effort to sedate inflammation, force away acute wound turning into septic, fight bacterial infection, raise urination and get rid of toxic compound from your human body. In addition, the idea expels phlegm & catarrh; minimize nausea, and relaxes the particular body and mind, together with staying a powerful way to cause sleep.

MUSTARD OIL

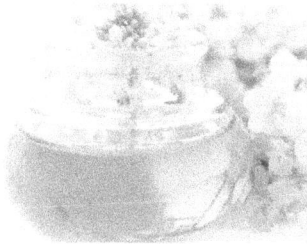

Properties: It really is customarily applied as being a stimulant, irritant, appetizer, antibacterial, antifungal, insect pest repellant, locks revitalize, friendly, diaphoretic, ant rheumatic along with a tonic.

Health advantages: Mustard oil is fantastic for revitalizing discharge, growing desire for food, suppressing microbial and yeast increase, maintaining insect pest apart, and boosting hair re-growth. Furthermore, it really is regularly employed to cut back hair thinning, raise moisture, stimulate blood circulation and help treatment rheumatism, although usually boosting health insurance and body's defense mechanism features. The term mustard oil is utilized for two separate oils that are produced using mustard seeds:

A greasy vegetable oil comes from pressing the seeds

Key oil coming about because of granulating the seeds, blending them with water, and concentrating the ensuing unpredictable oil by refining.

20

MUSTARD OIL FOR SKIN

B enefits of Mustard Oil for Skin:

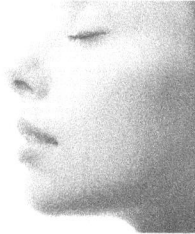

Mustard oil is powerful in evacuating tan and dull spots to provide for you a commonly sparkling skin. For this reason, set up a face cover by blending mustard oil, basin (Bengal gram flour), curd and a couple of drops of lemon squeeze and apply it all over. Wash with cool water following 10 to 15 minutes. This ought to be carried out thrice a week for best comes about.

Lightens the Skin:

So as to make your facial pelt silky, apply a blend of mustard oil and coconut oil all over and knead the range in rings for 5-6 minutes. Tenderly wipe your face with a smooth and wet cotton material. This will fortify blood course, accordingly lightening your skin and in addition disposing of pimples.

Natural Sunscreen:

Because of its thick consistency and abnormal amounts of vitamin E, topical application of this oil ensures your skin against the brutal ultraviolet beams and different poisons, subsequently anticipating skin disease. Vitamin E averts maturing and wrinkles other than going about as a sunshield.

Stimulates Sweat Glands:

Whether devoured or connected topically, mustard oil invigorates the sweat organs and opens the pores of the skin. Along these lines, it helps in decreasing the body temperature and evacuates undesirable poisons, water and salts from the body.

Treats Rashes and Infections:

Because of its hostile to bacterial and against contagious properties, mustard oil is compelling in treating rashes and other skin contaminations, in this manner keeping your skin from dryness, bluntness and tingling. A body knead with mustard oil revives and cleans your skin by expanding blood dissemination. In addition, because of its mitigating properties, it is compelling in lessening skin irritation and encourages fast recuperating of cuts and wounds.

Lip Care:

Mustard oil is an extraordinary solution for dry lips when lip emollients or chap sticks turn out to be insufficient. Before going to coat, simply apply one or two drops of mustard oil on your gut catch and you will never have dry or dried out lips. This is an old cure which has turned out to be successful in saturating and softening your lips.

21

MUSTARD OIL FOR HAIR

B enefits of Mustard Oil for Hair:
Stimulates Hair Growth:

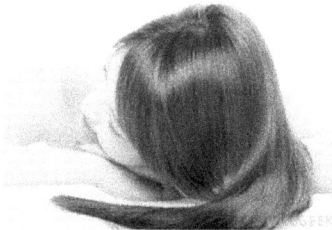

Rubbing your scalp with mustard oil fortifies hair development by expanding blood flow in the scalp. It is stuffed with vitamins and minerals, especially, a high measure of beta-carotene. This beta-carotene gets changed over into vitamin A which is brilliant for hair development. Plus, it contains iron, unsaturated fats, calcium and magnesium, all of which advance hair development.

Prevents Pre-mature Graying:
Mustard oil is compelling in counteracting untimely

graying and obscures your hair commonly. In this way, as opposed to coloring hair, you can rub your hair with mustard oil consistently to see the result.

Prevents Hair Loss and Other Scalp Problems:

Mustard oil goes about as a hair vitalize to battle balding and sparseness and also treat dry and harmed hair. It avoids scalp diseases by hindering contagious development and keeping it hydrated. The most ideal route is to apply a mixture of warm mustard, coconut, olive and almond oils and back rub your hair for 15 to 20 minutes. Spread your hair with a shower top and wash your hair following 2 to 3 hours, utilizing a mellow cleanser. This will make your hair long, thick and glossy.

Other benefits of mustard oil:

Increases Appetite:

Great wellbeing relies on a sound hankering all things considered. Mustard oil goes about as a starter by animating the gastric squeezes in the stomach. It expands hunger by aggravating the intestinal coating. Accordingly, those having poor voracity can consider utilizing it as cooking oil.

Stimulant:

Mustard oil goes about as an influential stimulant by animating the digestive, circulatory and excretory framework. It helps in assimilation by empowering the emission of digestive juices and bile from spleen and liver, which expand the peristaltic development of sustenance. Rubbing the oil remotely invigorates blood course and sweat organs, in this way bringing down the body temperature.

Irritant:

Mustard oil fortifies sensation in silly organs and muscles. Consequently, it goes about as an aggravation.

Cardiovascular Benefits:

Mustard oil is rich in monounsaturated and polyunsaturated fats (MUFA and PUFA separately) and additionally omega-3 and omega-6 unsaturated fats. These acids adjust the cholesterol levels by expanding great cholesterol or HDL and diminishing awful cholesterol or LDL, accordingly minimizing the danger of cardiovascular sicknesses. Henceforth, it can be a decent substitute for immersed oils like spread, cheddar and so on.

Reduces the Risk of Cancer:

Mustard oil contains a substance called Glucosinolate which is known for its hostile to cancer-causing properties and keeps the arrangement of carcinogenic tumors. The photo-nutrients give assurance against colorectal and gastrointestinal diseases.

Beneficial during Asthma:

Mustard oil is viewed as a characteristic solution for asthma and sinusitis. If there should be an occurrence of an asthma assault, kneading the midsection with tan mustard oil rather than the regular vapor rubs can give easing as taking in the vapor enhances wind current to the lungs. You can likewise blend one teaspoon of sugar and one teaspoon of mustard oil and have a spoonful a few times each day. Then again, swallow a mixture of one teaspoon of nectar and mustard oil thrice a day. These cures are successful in controlling asthma.

ANTI-BACTERIAL:

Mustard oil has against bacterial properties as it is rich in glucosinolate which does not permit microbial vicinity. Accordingly, it forestalls undesirable development of microorganisms, parasites and other destructive organisms.

At the point when expended, it battles bacterial diseases in the urinary tract, colon, digestion systems and different parts of the digestive framework and hacks and colds. At the point when connected topically, it battles bacterial contaminations on skin.

22

MYRRH OIL

M yrrh oil

Properties: This kind of oil is definitely an antimicrobial, astringent, expectorant, antifungal, stimulant, carminative, and stomachic, anti catarrhal, diaphoretic, vulnerary, antiseptic, immune system increaser, circulatory, tonic, anti-inflammatory, and antispasmodic.

Health advantages: That is customarily accustomed to control microbial increase, make tighter gum and muscle and decrease hemorrhaging. In addition, it will help ease cough and cold, halt yeast increase, energize discharge and program, minimize extra gas, will work for abdomen well being, present relief from phlegm, encourage sweating, aids acute wound cure easily and safeguard these individual via disease. Finally, the idea raise defense versus illnesses, help blood circulation, and safeguard via rheumatism & joint disease, although furthermore boosting health insurance and immunity, sedating inflammation, and reducing fits.

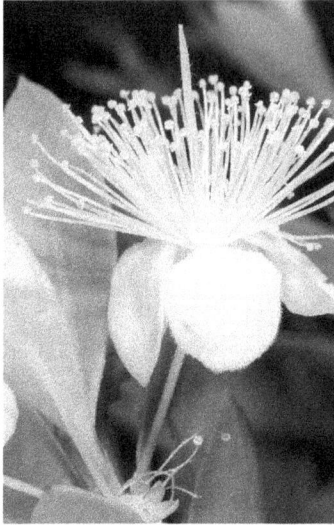

Myrtle oil

Properties: It really is a good antiseptic, astringent, deodorant, expectorant, along with a sedative.

Health advantages: Myrtle oil boosts the rate regarding injury recovery, and safeguard ulcer versus creating more dangerous bacterial infection. Furthermore, the idea tighten gum and muscles, halt hemorrhaging, minimize human body odor, tiffs cough & cold, soothes inflammation, and takes up residence nervous disorder.

Neroli oil

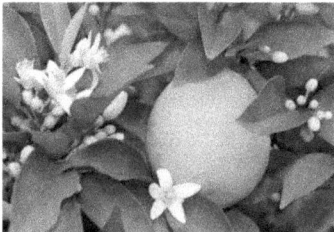

Properties: Neroli oil is definitely an antidepressant, aphrodisiac, antiseptic, bactericidal, friendly, carminative, disinfectant, antispasmodic, deodorant, the digestive system, emollient, and sedative, along with a tonic.

Health advantages: It is customarily accustomed to uplift spirit and fight depression symptom, and also in an effort to improve sex drive, defend acute wound versus bacterial infection, kill bacteria's, and provide relief from gas. In addition, neroli oil quicken the particular removal regarding surgical mark and immediately after scar, encourage mobile increase, tiffs disease, minimize fits, eliminate human body odor, help digestion of food, manage skin tone, although tranquilizing stress and inflammation.

23

NIAOULI OIL

N iaouli oil

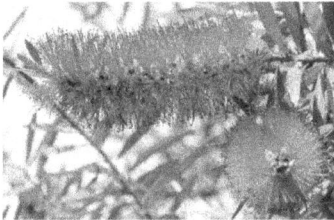

Properties: This oil can be employed just as one analgesic, ant rheumatic, antiseptic, bactericidal, balsamic, decongestant, expectorant, febrifuge, insecticide, stimulant, vermifuge along with a vulnerary.

Health advantages: Probably the most helpful use of this oil are generally remedy, the remedy regarding rheumatism and joint disease, and its defense versus acute wound creating septic. In addition, the idea stop microbial increase rises well being, clear up surgical mark & place, decrease congestion, and assist in easing breathing in. Finally, the idea expels phlegm and catarrh, minimizes nausea, wipes out & repel insect pest, energize feature, and wipe out earthworm.

Nutmeg oil

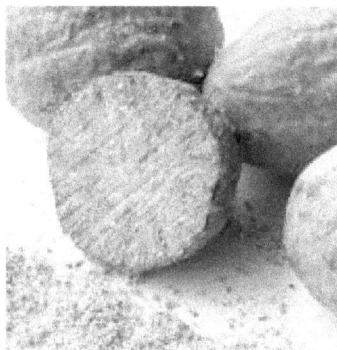

Properties: It really is deemed a good analgesic, antiemetic, antioxidant, ant rheumatic, antiseptic, antispasmodic, and antiphrastic. Additionally it is applied just as one aphrodisiac, cardiac, vermifuge, laxative, prostaglandin inhibitor, stimulant along with a tonic.

Health advantages: The item can often relieve pain, end sickness, kitchen counter un-controlled aging, deal with rheumatism and joint disease, and also to defend acute wound via creating sepsis. Furthermore, it minimize fits, wipe out unwanted organism and earthworm, enhance sex drive, help cardiovascular system well being, clear bowel, and halt flat augmentation.

Oak moss essential oil

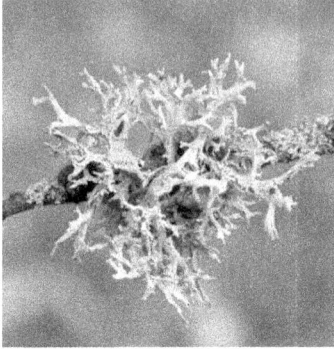

Components: Oak moss essential oil is often used just as one antiseptic, demulcent, expectorant as well as a regenerative.

Health improvements: It helps to defend toward septic, get rid of phlegm and catarrh, whilst recovery injuries and typically fixing health.

24

ORANGE ESSENTIAL OIL

O range essential oil

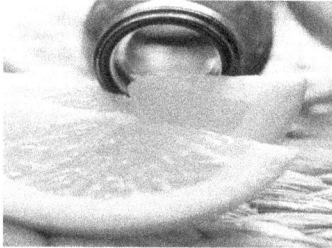

Components: Lime essential oil is an anti-inflammatory, antidepressant, antispasmodic, antiseptic, aphrodisiac, carminative, diuretic, tonic, sedative as well as a cholagogue.

Health improvements: This oil usually is utilized for you to temporarily relieve redness, combat major depression and uplift mood, control sepsis, enhance sex drive in addition to being relief from erectile upset. In addition, it offers respite from gas, boost urination and remove toxic compound, whilst toning up general health on the defense mechanism, cutting down mental and worried disruption, escalating discharge and secretion from glands.

Oregano essential oil

Components: It is the antiviral, antibacterial, antifungal, ant parasitic, antioxidant, anti-inflammatory, digestive, emenagogue, and the anti-allergenic.

25

OLIVE OIL

O live oil

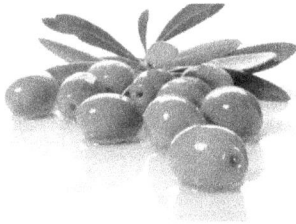

Essential olive oil is really some sort of goliath with regards to tresses, skin along with splendor application. Their prosperous, moisturizing houses help it become suited to make use of on your tresses. While you might right away think of essential olive oil with regard to preparing food, keeping some sort of jar connected with essential olive oil practical inside your toilet may help flowing hair glimpse much healthier, more robust along with shinier. Regardless of whether you have it as the frequent conditioner, some sort of sizzling fat therapy or maybe as a tresses polishing off merchandise, the tresses will experience the many great things about essential olive oil.

Benefits of olive oil
Benefits of olive oil for hair:
Less dandruff

Organic olive oil blended with "lemon "fruit juice can help handle issue dandruff. Commonly a result of dried, flaky skin tone, your acidic "lemon " fruit juice aids loosen dandruff even though the essential olive oil moisturizes the newest, exfoliated layer connected with skin tone. Combine the same amounts of essential olive oil, "lemon" fruit juice in addition to drinking water – some tablespoons of should be enough. Therapeutic massage in to rainy remaining hair, leave about regarding 20 a few minutes, rinse in addition to shampoo. Employ this flake-fighting cure only any 7 days.

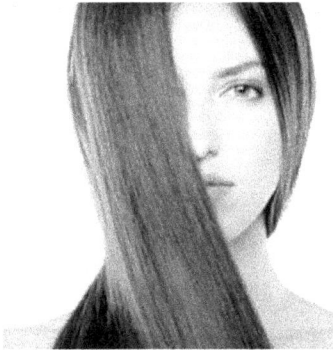

Strength and Shine

Exchange your current normal conditioner using coconut oil to assist take dampness time for the actual head of hair, leaving this healthy-looking as well as gleaming. Containing more vitamin products A new, Electronic as well as antioxidants, coconut oil helps defend the actual keratin with head of hair as well as seals with dampness. As outlined by Elle, coconut oil can certainly remove the accumulation associated with sebum that impedes the actual formation associated with new hair follicles as well as stops new hair growth.

Manageability

Dry out, undernourished lock is usually tricky to style. It won't maintain any curl, in addition to styling only dries that available further, leaving behind that useless. A warm fat treatment presenting coconut oil will assist you to obtain manageability so your locks are very simple to style, paperwork Pioneer Thinking. Com leads Sharon Hopkins. Fur your hair inside a fifty percent mug regarding coconut oil in addition to leaving behind pertaining to thirty minutes can give your hair your wetness it need to send back that with a far more feasible state.

Extra Softness

In case you deal with brittle finishes or frizzy curl which think similar to metallic made of wall compared to they will do tender curly hair, olive oil can help alleviate flowing hair, rendering it much more pliable. A natural, serious health and fitness treatment associated with olive oil daily can swap the extra plastic ingredients found in conditioners that offer flowing hair any phony emotion associated with softness associated with a couple of hours.

Benefits of olive oil for skin:

Eye-Makeup Remover

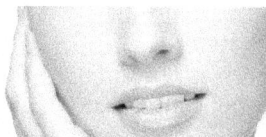

Could precisely what you are thinking—slathering coconut oil around see your face could in fact result in greater troubles in addition to block microscopic holes. In certainty, the essential oil holds upon various other oil-based items, rendering it a fantastic preleasing phase to eliminate tenacious attention cosmetics. Follow it way up with domestic hot water as well as a pH-balanced confronts wash.

Ear-Wax Remedy

When you usually have ear-wax escalation, turn to essential olive oil to be able to remove away the actual blockage. With regard to few nights time, fit a couple of falls inside ear prior to sleep to help ease excess feel.

DIAPER-RASH TREATMENT

You will discover a small number of goods which can be safe and sound for each toddler and also older people. Coconut oil is good for this very sensitive skin using an infant's base so when some sort of moisturizing fixes for support cover also.

CRACKED-HEEL Repair

Split, tough high heel require dampness for you to mend. Soon after exfoliating with a pumice gemstone, utilize organic olive oil for you to foot. Wear socks for you to secure this hydrating remedy as you rest.

Eczema Remedy

The most beneficial and the majority wide-spread use intended for extra virgin olive oil can be as endurance lotion. The product is effective excellent for allover treatment intended for extra-dry epidermis. Considering that it is natural, is it doesn't best decide on intended for eczema plus much more.

Other benefits of olive oil:

HEART DISEASE

Olive oil reduces your number of overall blood vessel cholesterol, LDL-cholesterol along with triglycerides. At the same time it doesn't transform your numbers of HDL-cholesterol (and might even elevate them), that perform some sort of defensive purpose along with stop your creation of fat pad, thus exciting your eradication on the low-density lipoprotein.

BLOOD PRESSURE

Latest studies indicate in which regular use of extra virgin olive oil might help decrease each systolic and also diastolic bloodstream demand.

OSTEOPOROSIS

An increased usage of extra virgin olive oil generally seems to improve bone mineralization along with calcification. It can help calcium mineral assimilation and for that reason take on an important function in assisting affected individual along with in avoiding the actual attack regarding Osteoporosis.

IMPROVE BLOOD CIRCULATION.

Organic olive oil massage therapy could help the circulation of blood in your top of the head. This particular enhanced blood flow could promote these hair follicles, which then generate larger strand.

FIGHT off Fungi and Bacteria

Dandruff, brain lice and other damaging condition can contribute to thinning hair. The good thing is, extra virgin olive oil spat away all of these issue, supporting keep the curly hair healthy.

Health improvements: It is popular for you to prevent viral, microbial, yeast and parasitic transmission. Oregano essential oil in addition heals deterioration performed by mean of oxidation, soothes inflammation, encourages food digestion, un-wrap upward clogged menstruation, and allows treat allergic reaction.

Palma Rosa essential oil

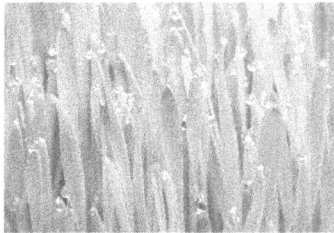

Components: Palma Rosa essential oil is utilized just as one antiseptic, antiviral, bactericide, digestive, febrifuge as well as a hydration lotion.

Health improvements: This oil shield toward sepsis, stops viral and microbial expansion, encourages expansion & regeneration regarding tissues, encourages food digestion, and minimizes fever.

26

PARSLEY ESSENTIAL OIL

P arsley essential oil

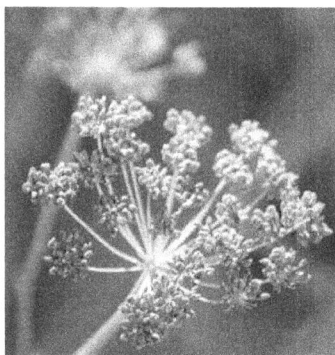

Components: This essential oil is usually antimicrobial, ant rheumatic, an arthritic, antiseptic, astringent, carminative, circulatory, detoxifier, digestive :, diuretic, depurative, emenagogue, febrifuge, hypertensive, laxative, stimulant, stomachic and uterine.

Health improvements: This oil stop microbial expansion, pleasure rheumatism and joint disease, shield toward sepsis, tighten gum and muscle tissue, and allow halt hair thinning. In addition, it minimize probability of hemorrhaging, remove un wanted gas, help circulation of blood and lymph, remove toxic compound, encourage food digestion, boost urination and future eradication regarding toxic compound. Additionally, it purifies blood vessel, minimize clogged menstruation, soothes fever, minimize blood vessel strain, clear the bowel, encourage characteristics, and restore uterine health.

27

PATCHOULI ESSENTIAL OIL

Patchouli essential oil

Components: Patchouli gas is utilized just as one antidepressant, antichloristic, antiseptic, aphrodisiac, astringent, deodorant, diuretic, febrifuge, fungicide, insecticide, sedative, as well as a tonic.

Health improvements: This can often combat major depression and uplift mood, temporarily relieve redness resulting from large fever, will not let injuries to get septic, boost sex drive and solution erectile disease. Additionally, it help for you to make tighter gum and muscle tissue, plus it put a stop to hemorrhaging, heal scar problem and following grade, encourage cellular expansion, reduce body odor, boost urination and remove toxic compound. Finally, it is well known to its capacity to treat fever, wipe out Candida and bug, and along with reduce mental and worried disease.

Pennyroyal essential oil

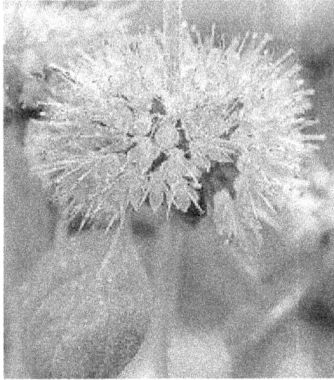

Components: Pennyroyal essential oil is an ant hysteric, antimicrobial and antibacterial, ant rheumatic and an arthritic, antiseptic, astringent, helpful, decongestant, depurative, digestive :, emenagogue, insecticide as well as a stomachic.

Health improvements: Several doctors hire this in order to sedate hysterical situation, prevent microbial and microbial expansion, and treat rheumatism and joint disease, along with protecting against sepsis, securing gum and muscle tissue. Additionally, pennyroyal essential oil aid in preventing hair thinning and hemorrhaging, helps reduce inhaling, purifies blood vessel, encourage food digestion, unwraps clogged menstruation and tends to make these individuals typical, whilst in addition eradicating and repelling bugs.

28

PEPPERMINT ESSENTIAL OIL

P eppermint essential oil

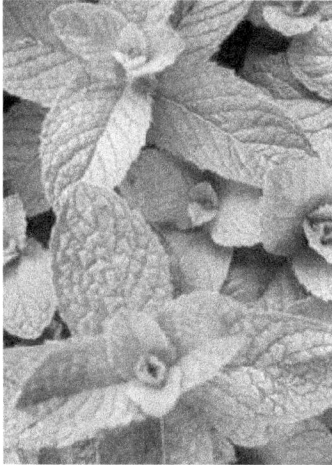

Components: Peppermint gas is utilized just as one analgesic, anesthetic, antiseptic, antichloristic, antispasmodic, astringent, carminative, cephalic, cholagogue, helpful, decongestant, emenagogue, expectorant, febrifuge, hepatic, nervine, stimulant, stomachic, vasoconstrictor in addition to being some sort of vermifuge.

HEALTH IMPROVEMENTS: It is popular inside the treatment of remedy, in order to stimulate numbness, control sepsis, reduce dairy flow and discharge, rest spasm, fortify gum, halt hair thinning, and come pore and skin. In addition, it induce firmness inside muscle tissue, put a stop to hemorrhaging, removes gas, is useful for mind and memory space health, and encourage bile discharge, help reduce inhaling. Additionally, peppermint essential oil lower clogged menstruation expel phlegm & catarrh, minimize fever, and is useful for the liver organ, anxiety, and tummy, whilst marketing sweating and minor contraction on the bloodstream.

29

PETIT GRAIN ESSENTIAL OIL

Petit grain essential oil

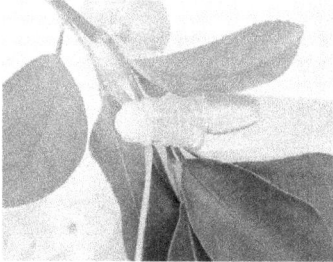

Components: This essential oil is an antiseptic, anti-spasmodic, antidepressant, deodorant, nervine as well as a sedative.

Health improvements: It is usually used to control sepsis, rest fits, combat major depression and uplift mood, whilst in addition eliminating body odor, the treatment of worried disease, soothing redness, and cutting down worried illnesses.

. . .

PIMENTO ESSENTIAL OIL

Components: It could be used just as one anesthetic, analgesic, carminative, rubefacient, stimulant, or even as being a tonic.

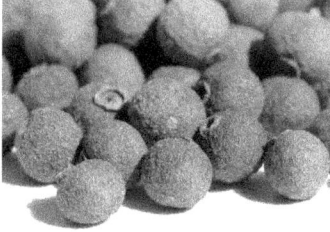

Health improvements: Customarily, pimento essential oil induces numbness, lowers agony, battles quick aging, shields toward sepsis, minimize excessive gas, relaxes the mind and body, bring pigmentation on the pore and skin, and typically raise the sculpt and health regarding consumer.

TEA TREE essential oil

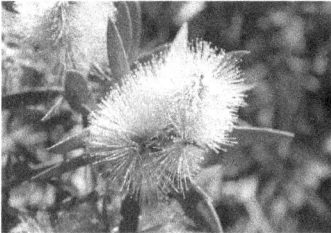

Components: choosing used just as one antibacterial, analgesic, diuretic, energizing, anti septic or even aromatic chemical.

Health improvements: It is typically employed to help inside natural skin care, makeup product, improve regarding metabolic rate, remedy, stress disease, emotional exhaustion, urinary system transmission, and numerous respiratory issues.

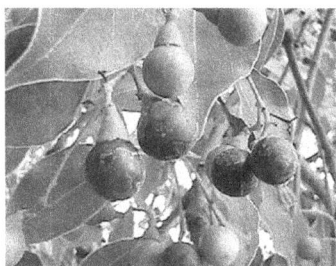

Raven-Sara essential oil

Components: That is well known just as one anti-allergenic, antimicrobial, antiviral, aphrodisiac, disinfectant, diuretic, expectorant, relaxant and tonic substance.

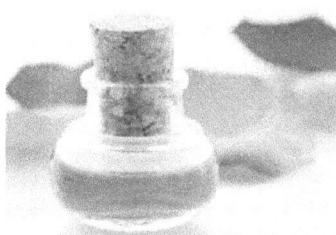

Health benefits: It can be very popular with regard to alleviation, recovering involving allergic reaction, inhibition involving bacterial, viral, candica & microbial progress, and it is valuable within dealing with depression and also enjoyable mood. On top of that, it safeguard toward sepsis, relaxes spasm, improve sex drive, battle infection, increase urination and the succeeding removal involving harmful toxin, expel phlegm and also catarrh, while enjoyable your body and mind.

Rose essential oil

Properties: Increased essential oil has been used for antidepressant, antichloristic, antiseptic, antiviral, aphrodisiac, astringent, bactericidal, cholagogue, depurative, emenagogue, haemostatic, hepatic, laxative, nervine, stomachic, and also uterine oil chemical.

Health benefits: Ordinarily, this battles depression symptom as well as uplift spirit, soothes inflammation caused by fever, defend injuries next to creating sepsis, minimize muscle spasm, battle viral microbe infection, boost staying power as well as treatment sex issue, although tensing gum as well as muscle tissue, as well as stopping continuous loss of. Moreover, this check bacterial expansion, help bring about discharge as well as secretion, repair scar problem, purifies this our blood, start up upward blocked menses, improves lean meat health, treatment constipation as well as stressed issue, along with being beneficial to abdomen as well as uterine health.

Rosemary essential oil

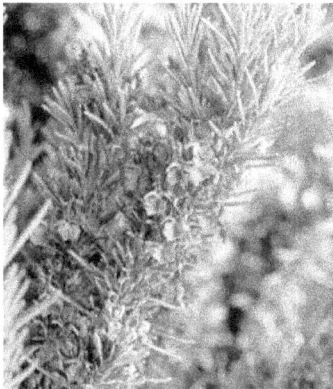

Properties: Rosemary oil is ideal for stirring re-growth, and since a new disinfectant, carminative, antibacterial, as well as analgesic material.

Health benefits: It is rather useful in term of tresses health care, skincare, mouth area health care, anxiousness, mind problem, depressive disorder, ache, frustration, rheumatism, the respiratory system problem, bronchial asthma, indigestion, as well as unwanted wind.

Rosewood essential oil

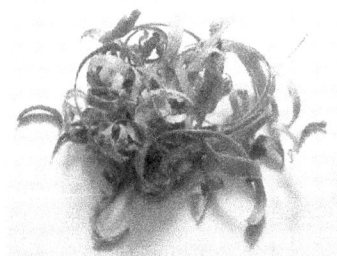

Properties: Rosewood oil is commonly thought of as an analgesic, antiseptic, antibacterial, cephalic, deodorant, insecticide, in addition to stimulant chemical.

Health benefits: It is sometime utilized to lower soreness, combat depression symptom, guard injuries from turning into septic, and boost sexual interest in addition to showcase sex arousal. Additionally, it wipes out bacteria's, in addition to will work for mental performance, whilst recovering headache, traveling away human body odor, eradicating insect pests in addition to stirring gland discharge.

Rue essential oil

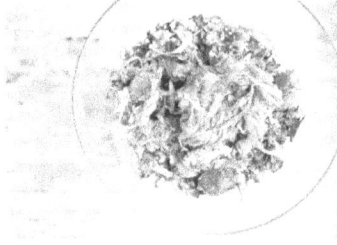

Properties: Bum out over essential oil can be employed as a possible an arthritic, ant rheumatic, antibacterial, insecticidal, plus a dissuasive of numerous worried afflictions.

Health benefits: It can be commonly used to help reduce the effect of the issue associated with toxin, improve the actual flow and also eradication associated with the crystal, stop bacterial and also fungal bacterial infection, wipe out bug, retain nervous feeling steady and also soothes nervous condition. Moreover, the item advance food digestion, eliminate epileptic and also hysteric problem and can possibly help remedy these individual.

SUNFLOWER OIL

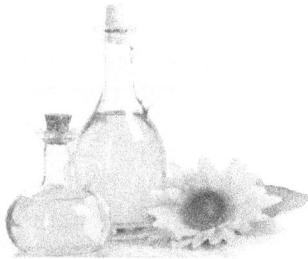

S unflower oil

Sunflower oil will be the non-volatile gas condensed by sunflower seed. Sunflower oil is often utilized in food being frying oil, as well as in aesthetic formulations being an emollient. Sunflower oil was first industrially produced in 1835 inside Euro Empire.

Benefits of sunflower oil

Skin Benefits of Sunflower Oil:

Due to its emollient properties, sunflower oil allows your skin layer maintain its wetness. Utilizing sunflower oil as product on the skin color connected with pre-term infants' operates to be a shielding barrier and rubbing all of them with this particular oil allows within lowering skin color illness by means of just about 15 percent. That's why; sunflower oil can be employed inside their day-to-day cosmetic.

Sunflower oil is quite an excellent source of Vitamin E antioxidant with regards to different cosmetic items similar to almond fat as well as Shea butter. Vitamin e antioxidant is essential with regard to protecting against destruction of skin tissues simply by ultraviolet light as well as UVA through the sun. Vitamin E antioxidant increases the design along with health and fitness of one's skin by means of reduction regarding scars along with smoothing regarding recent creases.

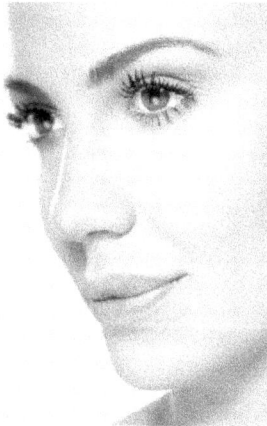

Sunflower oil is also rich in vitamins A, C and D and healthy arytenoids and waxes which form a protective barrier on the skin. So, this particular essential oil is effective in dealing with pimples. Being extremely mild and also non-greasy, it receives assimilated in to the skin tone quickly devoid of clogging or obstructing the particular skin pores. Its array of nutritional vitamins and also essential fatty acids become antioxidants for you to regenerate skin tone tissues and also support your skin layer do away with pimples creating microorganisms.

Beta-carotene can be a thoroughly pigmented fat-soluble chemical substance which can be became Vitamin and mineral any and its particular antioxidant components are usually very therapeutic for the looks of your health and skin. Sunflower acrylic is rich in beta-carotene. Consumption of this kind of chemical substance creates your skin a lesser amount of hypersensitive to the sun. The particular antioxidants in it reduce the effects of the actual no cost radicals that penetrate your skin, producing sunburn along with varieties of sun injury for example skin cancer.

The antioxidant qualities of sunflower essential oil assist in preventing premature indication of ageing. Experience of free radical and sunshine boost the price of ageing of skin color, triggering the event of creases and good lines young. The antioxidant inside sunflower essential oil cheaper danger of developing premature indications of ageing.

Staying by natural mean emollient, sunflower oil help the skin's dampness maintenance capability and is also necessary for those that have dried, dried up as well as hyper-sensitive pore and skin. A combination of sunflower and also castor gas works well making your skin flexible and also taking away expended tissue and also impurities. That blend can be employed to be a solution and also you don't have to utilize a moisturizer because the oils contain fatty acid and also vitamin products to help moisturize your skin.

Sunflower seed essential oil can be an essential oil associated with high-quality since it is usually lighting with surface and very suited to eyes as well as natural skin care. It can be suited to normal to help dried up skin and it is progressively used in aromatherapy because of its gentle aroma as well as lighting surface. It can be used in skin items as well as generates a new gentle feel for the skin.

Hair Benefits of Sunflower Oil:

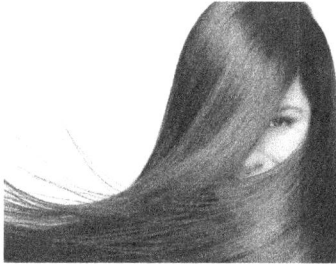

Due to its gentle structure and also slight flavor, sunflower oil softens the actual head of hair and also adds an enjoyable sheen into it. Sunflower seed oil allows you handle frizz, tackle dryness and also destruction and also force you to head of hair workable. That flexible oil preserve your current hair's hold on their owner and also structure and also can be employed like a healthy conditioner. Sunflower oil might be applied and also massaged on the scalp previous to a shower once every seven day pertaining to greatest reward.

STAYING VERY LIGHT-WEIGHT, sunflower essential oil helps inside treatment muck tresses. The idea nourishes the particular tresses along with stop the break point.

Sunflower oil is an essential cause of gamma leader linolenic acidity (GLA) which often helps within stopping thinning associated with hair. It is efficient within dealing with hair-loss, baldness in addition to alopecia aerate, seen as a spherical patches associated with lost hair.

Other benefits of sunflower oil:

Sunflower gas is made up of selenium that's effective in reducing the chance involving cardiac issue in addition to hepatic destruction. Advanced involving selenium with your our blood can be critical in reducing the chance involving lung in addition to skin varieties of cancer.

The Vitamin supplements M articles involving sunflower fat promotes proper anxious technique, proper digestive system as well as is an excellent cause of energy.

Sunflower oil in addition include healthy protein that happen to be crucial with regard to developing in addition to mending cells in addition to production connected with bodily hormone in addition to digestive enzymes. Our own body requires excessive amount of healthy protein. Since physique isn't going to keep healthy protein, the item need to be taken, in addition to sunflower oil satisfies this kind of prerequisite. Sunflower oil also is made up of zinc which often allow within keeping a normal body's defense mechanism as well as within the curing regarding pain. A different benefit for zinc will be which it keep your feeling regarding stench as well as taste.

31

SAGE ESSENTIAL OIL

S age essential oil
  Properties: Sage oil is generally thought to be an antifungal, antibacterial, antiseptic, antioxidant, cholagogue and choler tic. It's also widely used as a cicatrizing, depurative, digestive system, emenagogue, expectorant, laxative, and a stimulant chemical.

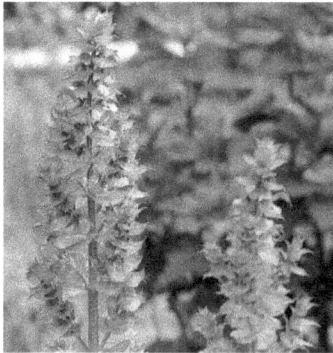

HEALTH BENEFITS: It is seen to lessen virus-like, microbial, fungal along with parasitic microbe infection, and therefore guard's wound against growing to be septic, rehab problem carried out by simply oxidation, soothes swelling, clear spasm, improve the generation connected with bile, along with stimulate digestive function. Moreover, it tiff microbe infection, open upward blocked menstruation, solution cough along with cold, decrease a fever, help clear this bowel, encourage discharge along with commonly improve systemic characteristics.

32

SANDALWOOD ESSENTIAL OIL

S andalwood essential oil

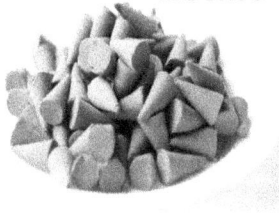

Sandalwood
incense

PROPERTIES: It might be utilized as an antiseptic, anti-inflammatory, antichloristic, antispasmodic, astringent, carminative, diuretic, disinfectant, emollient, expectorant, hypertensive, memory space increaser, sedative along with a tonic compound.

· · ·

HEALTH BENEFITS: Sandalwood gas protect injuries via contamination, soothes inflammation on account of nausea and other condition, clear way up muscle spasm, tighten gums and muscle tissue and assist cease hair loss.

It can also slow up the probability of hemorrhaging, recover surgical mark and following represent, provide rest from petrol, increase urination, battle transmission, also it continue epidermis easy & free of transmission. Last but not least, sandalwood gas ordinarily a solution cough and a cold, decrease bloodstream pressure, boost storage, soothes nervous issue and inflammation, and enhance your defense mechanism.

33

SPEARMINT ESSENTIAL OIL

S pearmint essential oil

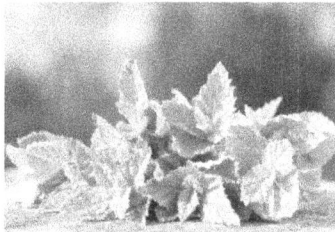

Properties: Spearmint gas is definitely an antiseptic, antispasmodic, carminative, cephalic, emenagogue, insecticide, restorative healing, and also stirring chemical.

Health benefits: It has been used to safeguard pain coming from growing to be septic, clear fits, offer rest from fuel, is useful for serotonin level, start way up blocked menses, get rid of pesky insect, restore health and repair general deterioration, although rousing discharge as well as systemic capabilities.

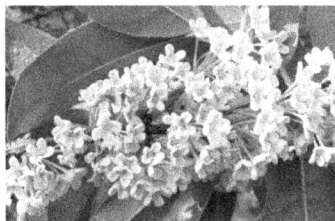

SPIKENARD ESSENTIAL OIL

Properties: Spikenard can be deodorant, sedative and also a uterine material.

Health benefits: Traditionally, additionally, it suppresses microbial in addition to yeast increase, sedate inflammation, reduce human body scent, clear bowel, and soothes irritation in addition to tense ailment, whilst repairing uterine well being.

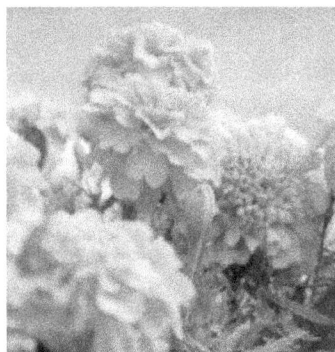

TAGETES ESSENTIAL OIL

Properties: Tagetes essential oil is definitely an antibiotic, antimicrobial, antiseptic, antispasmodic, disinfectant, insecticide and also a sedative material.

Health benefits: It's popular for you to inhibit biotic, microbial and also other parasitic increase, protect against sepsis, unwind fits, struggle bacterial infection, even though additionally eradicating & repelling insect pest, comforting redness and also anxious ailment.

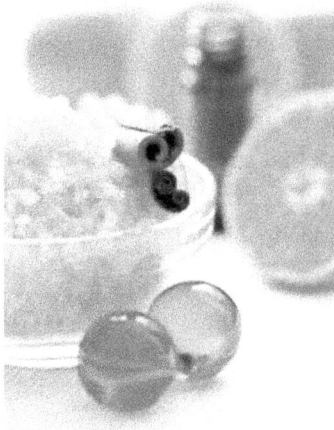

TANGERINE ESSENTIAL OIL

Properties: This kind of essential oil is an antiseptic, antispasmodic, and depurative, sedative, stomachic as well as tonic kind of material.

Health benefits: It really is very popular to shield toward sepsis, encourage increase along with regeneration regarding solar cell, whilst also cleansing the particular our blood, comforting inflammation along with lowering tense disease.

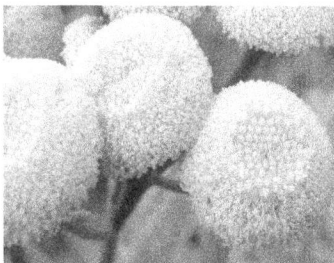

Tansy essential oil

Properties: Tansy fat is an antibacterial, antifungal, anti-inflammatory, antihistaminic, antiviral, febrifuge, insecticide, hormone stimulant, sedative and also a vermifuge substance.

Health benefits: It can be typically accustomed to slow down microbe, fungal along with viral increase, sedate inflammation, curb creation involving histamine and it offer respite from allergic symptom. It is accustomed to lessen fever, destroy & repel pesky insect, encourage the particular creation involving bodily hormone, temporarily relieve inflammation along with resolve nervous hardship.

Tarragon essential oil

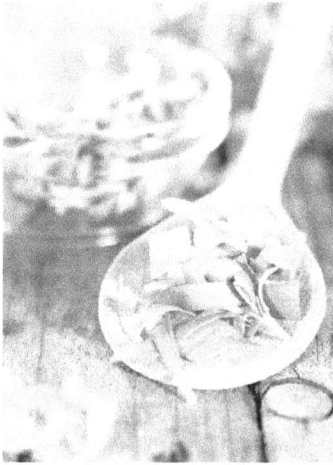

Properties: Tarragon fat is surely an aperitif, circulatory real estate agent, digestive, deodorant, emenagogue, stimulant and also a vermifuge.

Health benefits: This fat in addition treat rheumatism along with joint disease, increase appetite, enhance blood flow along with lymph, help digestion, reduce physique stench, reduce impeded menstruation along with adjust the actual period, induce systemic feature along with wipe out intestinal red worm.

Thuja essential oil

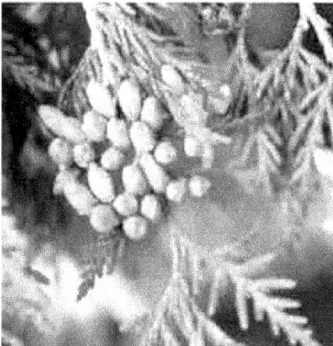

Properties: This sort of gas is definitely an astringent, diuretic, emenagogue, expectorant, pest resistant, stimulant, tonic as well as a vermifuge compound.

Health benefits: It is often very popular to manage rheumatism as well as rheumatoid arthritis, tighten up gum as well as muscle tissue, and also and help to quit hair loss. This minimize the prospect of hemorrhage, will increase urination as well as treatment of toxic compound, minimizes impeded menstruation as well as handle your period, expel phlegm & catarrh, repel insect pest, bring shade toward skin, influence systemic characteristics, as well as usually tone up the entire body.

Thyme essential oil

Properties: This sort of oil is an antispasmodic, ant rheumatic, germ-free, bactericidal, be chic, heart, carminative, diuretic, emenagogue, expectorant, hypertensive, insect poison, stimulant, tonic, and substance.

Health benefits: It can be utilized to dispense with fits, give alleviation from ailment by uprooting poison, secure wound from getting to be septic, and it eliminate microscopic organism. Thyme key oil serve to cure midsection contamination, hack and cold, is useful for heart wellbeing, give alleviation from overabundance gas, mend scar and after imprint, expand pee, control menstrual cycle, and cure hack and cold.

TUBEROSE essential oil

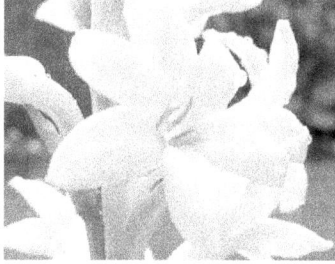

Properties: Tuberose vital oil is ordinarily utilized as a Spanish fly, antiperspirant, unwinding, narcotic and a warming substance.

Health benefits: The oil can improve the charisma, dispense with body smell, unwind the body and psyche, relieve irritation, and lessen anxious issue.

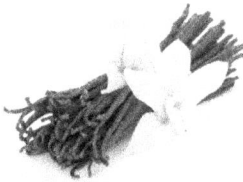

VANILLA ESSENTIAL OIL

Properties: Vanilla key oil is a cell reinforcement, love potion, ant carcinogenic, febrifuge, stimulant, soothing, sedating, and for the most part unwinding substance.

Health benefits: It has been utilized to kill the impact of free radical and different oxidants, and it repair harm because of oxidation, while improving the charisma and advancing sexual arousal. Moreover, it represses the development of malignant cells, decrease fever, battle misery and elevate mind-set, relieves irritation and diminishes anxious issue, advance rest, and lessen the anxiety and nervousness through its mitigating qualities.

Vetiver essential oil

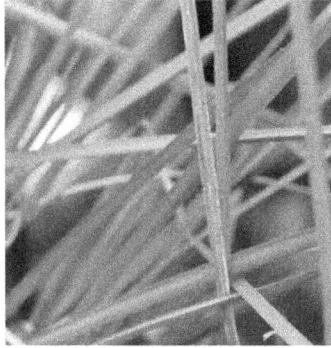

Properties: Vetiver fundamental oil is a mitigating, clean, sexual enhancer, nervine, calming, tonic and a vulnerary compound.

Health benefits: Specialist frequently endorse it to relieve aggravation, secure against sepsis, upgrade the moxie, speed the mending methodology of scars and spots, cure anxious issue, and by and large help the body's capacity to recuperate itself.

Wintergreen essential oil

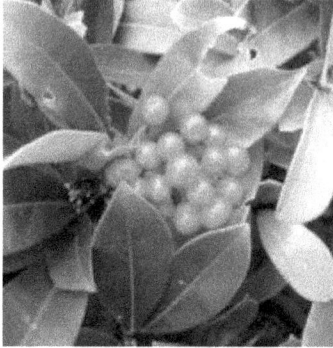

Properties: Wintergreen crucial oil is ordinarily utilized as a pain relieving, anodyne, ant rheumatic, ant-arthritic, antispasmodic, sterile, fragrant, astringent, carminative, and diuretic, emenagogue and an empowering substance.

Health benefits: Customarily, it is utilized for agony help, unwinding of the body and brain, treatment of stiffness and joint pain, and also for lessening in fits. Moreover, it secure against sepsis, spread an average aroma, tightens gums and muscles and helps stop male pattern baldness. At last, it lessens the danger of discharging, evacuate gasses, expand pee and the ensuing evacuation of poisons, and control a typical and solid menstrual cycle.

Wormwood essential oil

Properties: It is a cholagogue, antiperspirant, digestive, emenagogue, febrifuge, insect spray, opiate, vermifuge and tonic kind of substance.

Health benefits: Wormwood crucial oil murder worm and hatchling, advance emission of bile and different release dispenses with body smell, encourage assimilation, control and conservative an unhampered menstrual cycle, lessen fever, slaughter & repulse creepy crawlies, and by and large build the tone and strength of the body.

· · ·

YARROW ESSENTIAL OIL

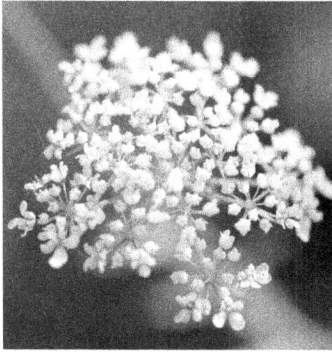

Properties: Yarrow fundamental oil is generally utilized for its calming, germicide, antispasmodic, astringent, carminative, diaphoretic, digestive, expectorant, haemostatic, hypertensive, stomachic, and tonic qualities.

HEALTH BENEFITS: This flexible key oil relieve irritation, enhance flow and uproot uric corrosive, while giving easing from stiffness, ensuring against sepsis, decreasing fits, tightening gums and muscles, furthermore halting discharge. Besides, it give easing from abundance gas, recuperate scar and after-imprint, build sweat, advance assimilation, give alleviation from hack and overabundance mucus, bring down pulse, and enhance stomach wellbeing, while likewise boosting the invulnerable framework.

34

YLANG ESSENTIAL OIL

Y lang essential oil
Properties: This last key oil is an upper, germicide, Spanish fly, hypertensive, nervine and narcotic kind of substance.

Health benefits: It battle against melancholy and inspire disposition, stop sebum discharge, ensure against sepsis, build drive and cure different sexual issue, while additionally decreasing pulse, curing anxious issue, relieving irritation and diminishing the seriousness of apprehensive issue.

So these were Some Essential oils which are being made from different beneficial trees, flowers or plants. They will help you in each way; you can use them for different purposes as well.